Getting Through Menopause

Solutions for Night Sweats, Hot Flashes and Weight Gain

By Haley Lynn

Requests for permission should be addressed to the GTM Permissions Department,
12018 Quito Rd Richmond VA 23112 or by email to Lyn8nn@gmail.com.

ISBN-13 978-1501034282 (paperback)

ISBN-10 1501034286

Printed in the United States of America

20 19 18 17 16 15 14 13 12 11 10 9 8 7 6 5 4

While the author has devoted many years to the acquisition of this information, there are no representations or warranties with respect to the accuracy or completeness of the contents of this book and specifically disclaims any implied warranties for infallibility of advice or fitness for a particular purpose. Knowledge and information increases every month; new information always supersedes old. This publication is designed to provide interesting and authoritative information in regard to the subject matter covered. Examples used in this book are altered to protect privacy. Please consult your doctor when circumstances are worrisome to you.

Table of Contents

Questions and Answers

No one knows it is menopause when it begins. We only see it in the rear view mirror. The start is never a day, or even a month. The symptoms aren't clear-cut enough. They fade in. Some of them appear to be something else. A missed period is thought to be pregnancy, and when it isn't, the incident falls from memory.

Dieting can cause a person to miss periods or increase the duration between periods. Travel, sleeping in strange beds or sitting next to other women for hours on trains and planes can also alter the menstrual cycle. Mostly, we think 'I'm too young' to be starting menopause, so we attribute symptoms to various causes.

Later on, for convenience and because the doctors ask, we'll have to pick a month sometime in the past and state that's when menopause started. It's the best we can do.

The first questions everyone has about menopause are, how long will it last? What can I do about the symptoms? What works? In just a few pages I'll get to those answers.

I debated with myself whether to talk about this first, middle or end of this book, and decided to mention it in the beginning.

There is a lot of baloney out there about menopause. There are many people trying to make a buck selling potions, supplements, treatments and diet plans to menopausal women. There may be some good ones mixed in with all the opportunist product hucksters; later on in this book I identify some known false claim products, plus some things that actually do work under certain circumstances.

If you're like me, this isn't the first book or article you're reading on menopause.

There's a lot of misinformation presented by people with a monetary interest in convincing you their treatment really works. Sadly, you're also going to read articles by well-meaning writers who just mash up several other articles from reputable sources and put it out there as fact.

I've seen articles in AARP's magazine that repeat the fallacies and misinformation in bullet-point fashion, as if they were absolutely true and no medical proof needed to be given.

Surprisingly, a far better source of information on what works and what doesn't is Consumer Reports. They don't take anyone else's statements for fact, no matter how many hundreds of times it's been said.

Far too much about menopause is written or stated by men. Where they got it from is hard to discern. I hope the information originally came from women, but I fear that often it is not the case.

There are three types of menopause writers to take with a grain of salt: first, medical people. They write books and articles treating it like a biology study. They deliver pages and pages on the workings of the thymus. They did the research so by golly they are going to write about it.

Realistically, no menopausal woman needs to know anything about the thymus. You don't need to be able to wire a house to flick a light switch. Reading up on how your innards work is as helpful to dealing with menopause as reading a book on car repair is to driving. You can be a good driver without knowing how fuel injection works, and you can handle menopause without learning about internal organs.

What is the average woman supposed to do with her new knowledge of the workings of a thymus anyway, or skin at the cellular level, or a thorough understanding of the effect of hormones on the vaginal skin?

These books are often thick. Helpful treatments are sometimes sprinkled in there, but the amount of reading it takes to collect them is almost not worth the effort.

These books simply overwhelm the reader with facts presented as if they are important, facts that are devoid of solutions. They cover every fringe and oddball situation, which is of dubious value unless you work in the medical field. If you're scientifically inclined and have lifelong interest in biology, they're fine. But couching them as mandatory reading for menopausal women is a bit of a stretch.

~ • ~

The second type are nearly always written by women. Women who have gone through menopause, so they know what they are talking about. They endeavor to make their readers feel good about being in menopause.

If the life-improving outlook and the morale-boosting words help, that is wonderful! I find some have an opposite effect, setting the bar too high for women with complicated lives. That leads to a sour feeling that menopause suffering is my own fault because I don't do what it takes to overcome the symptoms.

In reality, many authors count on almost no one fully implementing every single bit of their advice for even six months, which keeps the truth that it doesn't work unexposed. The more unworkable it is, the more it might be true, right?

They sound so convincing that eating healthy foods, getting on an exercise regimen, take herbal supplements, meditation, and so on is the way to weather menopause.

If the solution to menopause symptoms was to eat more green vegetables, we wouldn't have menopause, we'd just reach the age of two salads per day. Can certain foods make symptoms worse? I'll concede that. Certain food and drink can make you become flushed, get irritable or ruin sleep, menopause or not.

Is the opposite therefore true, are there foods that will cure menopause? If so, we'd have grown up knowing about them.

The reason the writers are so convinced is . . . this is their plan and they didn't have bad symptoms. The severity of menopausal symptoms is inherited. About 20% to 40% of women inherit few or mild menopausal symptoms. I'm happy for them. But they didn't stumble upon the cure in the produce aisle of the grocery store, no matter what they think.

If these things really worked three generations ago, twenty generations ago, even in the 1950s, they would simply be part of our culture, like eating fruit to prevent scurvy or taking in sunlight to prevent rickets.

~ • ~

The last group is the out-and-out make-a-buck guys. They hook you in with a plausible theory and very convincing stories and testimonials, and halfway through the book, infomercial, or magazine article, it morphs into a commercial for the product they're selling.

The testimonials are fake. Good-looking people are paid to do those, and paid to deny being paid.

Menopause treatments are the perfect scam. Placebo effect will make a small percentage of people feel it really helped them. All the customers are getting a little better every month whether they take anything or not.

If they can make you take their product for six months, your symptoms will be better simply because it's six months later. Even better, in six years, 80% of all customers have aged out of hot flashes entirely. Where's the legal case?

Any product which produces only a gradual, accumulative effect is not working at all. That gradual effect is simply you proceeding along the normal course.

Most of these products play it so coy on the labels and get so tricky with statements in printed material that they don't actually promise to relieve menopausal symptoms–not in the way the courts need to prove false claims.

If you are one of those who inherit a tendency for severe symptoms, you'll have hot flashes and really suffer. Doctors don't get it. Your friends don't get it.

It's not just the hot flash itself, but the waiting, never knowing when it will happen again. Half of the bad things attributed to menopause sound like the result of not getting enough sleep. This book will help you diminish waking up at night. If you get a night sweat, it will provide means to shorten the duration and get back to sleep. Getting enough sleep plays a huge part in weathering menopause with the least damage to your relationships with friends and family.

Talk to a woman about going through menopause. A woman older than you. It really, really helps. Menopause is like being pregnant, in that when you mention it, people who have done it before you freely share their own stories. When your head is in that place, those stories are enthralling.

It's hard to describe the warm feeling of true connection you get when women who have been merest acquaintances share their experience with menopause. Whether mild or severe, they all provide insight and information. Just becoming aware of the range of experience puts yours into perspective. It's easy to feel victimized. When you hear their stories, you will know you are not alone.

Reading it in a book is one thing, but hearing it from women you know is camaraderie. Make efforts to talk to women family members.

The clearest answer on how long hot flashes will last for you, how severe they are, and what kind of night sweats you'll have comes from asking your mother and her sisters plus your Dad's sisters, even asking older cousins what their experience was. Their experience is a bellweather to your path.

~ • ~

There's an old saying: Suspense is the life of a spider. You're living that spider life right now. Waiting for the next one to happen shadows daily life.

It's like living your life with a clown holding one of those big inflatable sharks standing right behind you and at random intervals –not even random, but picking the worst possible times—he starts bopping you on the head with it for ten minutes straight.

It won't leave a bruise and when you tell anyone how miserable it is, they laugh and accuse you of overreacting. It's hardly noticeable, they fib.

There's nothing you can do to get that clown to stop following you . . . night and day.

Randomly ruining your concentration, waking you up, causing every head to turn, making you cross and irritable . . . even when he isn't doing it, he's standing there like Chinese water torture ready to do it again at some interval he picks.

You feel like you're living on borrowed time until the next one. It feels like a shell of a life. And no one will bluntly and flat out tell you how long it will last. When will that clown be GONE?

~ • ~

Here's the answer to how long the miserableness of hot flashes / night sweats will last.

Most people notice night sweats before hot flashes start, although they might initially attribute it to just being too warm at night. Night sweats are first to come and last to leave.

A significant percentage of people have no daytime hot flashes but suffer terribly from night sweats.

For those getting daytime hot flashes, the severe ones with chills will last two years. The worst will peak about one to 1.5 years after the very first signs, which could be six months prior to the month you conclude this is in fact menopause. As time goes on the frequency will diminish. There will be more time between them, but when they come they'll be just as bad.

After more time, not only will they spread out but the severity will diminish. For half the women with hot flashes, the daytime hot flash intensity diminishes to tolerable by the third year, but they still have night sweats for several more years, getting steadily milder.

For some people hot flashes may wax and wane, meaning start, then another menstrual period commences so they disappear for a few weeks, then return. This come-and-go aspect makes the randomness more infuriating.

The chills that come after the hot flash are considered worse than the hot flash by many women. The chills are caused not only the coldness that sets in because one is wet, but something extremely uncomfortable and deeper, to the bone. This is a singularly uncomfortable stage that manifests shortly after the hot flash subsides and it lasts for several minutes.

Some have a few reduced-intensity daytime hot flashes into the fifth to eighth year. Sometime between six and ten years it will diminish down to ordinary life, mildly perceptible or perhaps totally gone.

Often it's simply that your standards are lowered, so you declare them over even when your temperature-regulating system is not as steady as it used to be.

Some women retain a nightly warmer spell or two that is sufficient, just barely, to wake them up. Some women are totally fed up with the clown by that time, so take a sleeping pill or potion to drown out awareness.

~ • ~

I'm disappointed with the medical community about their stonewall reluctance to talk about how hot flashes start out hot and heavy and then diminish. One would think they are in cahoots with the supplement scammers because they won't state firmly and without equivocation that getting 20% better over four months does not mean anything, that would have happened without spending any money. Time marches on, and it's time, not the pricey pill, that does it.

If you have a technique or product that really helps you, write an Amazon review to tell me about it. I'll be reading those and incorporating all your good suggestions in future revisions of this book. If your name is in your review, I'll credit you for the contribution. It's understandable if some people don't really want their fifteen minutes of fame to be related to a creative use of a juice box, or to menopause, so be sure to note whether you want your name used, want only your handle to be used, or wish to remain anonymous.

Hot flashes will happen more predictably when under stress, when you get a shock or startle, and even when laughing hard. Depending upon your skin color, they may not be noticeable to anyone but you, even if you are speaking before a crowd.

I myself wasn't so lucky; I flushed red each time for over seven years. A hot flash started when I heard a racy joke, when I was a tiny bit stressed, even when I suddenly realized I hadn't called back a friend I promised I would call back . . . every little thing made me flush.

I was saddled with an unwarranted reputation for being a touchy prude. It was partly my fault, because I'd just started a new job and refused to admit at work that I was having hot flashes. I wanted to retain the impression of being in my forties . . . in hindsight a big mistake.

There is a chapter in this book, *Tell or Not Tell?* That discusses the pros and cons of sharing, deciding what level of revelation makes sense in your life. This is actually a big deal, and you need to have a plan.

Prescribed hormone supplements are the only true fix. They basically fool your body into thinking you haven't reached menopause yet. Meaning they stave off menopause to a later date.

Even if your doctor will prescribe that medicine this year, at some point he or she is going to cut you off and tell you it's time to take your turn in the menopause barrel. Here comes the clown . . .

Hot Flashes & Night Sweats

All hot flashes, whether during the day or at night in bed, start on the back, between the shoulder blades. When this area gets too warm, it becomes one of the possible triggers for a hot flash to start. Keeping the area between the shoulder blades cool is the key to reducing the frequency of hot flash onset.

Cooling this area after the hot flash has started will prevent or significantly minimize the chills that follow hot flashes. Chills follow a hot flash for several months, possibly as long as two years. After that, hot flashes reduce in severity enough so the chill isn't that noticeable.

Some women have hot flashes only at night. One of the largest factors in menopause miserableness is being robbed of sleep. Whether you were a good sleeper before or woke up often, the good times are over. The clown is playing his shark-bopping game 24-7. You need techniques for getting through the night.

Emotional perfection will not eliminate hot flashes. A perfect diet will not eliminate hot flashes. Training for the Boston Marathon will not eliminate hot flashes. Things that help a bit do not mean that doubling those efforts results in half as many hot flashes.

What eliminates hot flashes is time. After the symptoms peak, it will be better six months later, and even better six months after that.

It might seem that cold chills stem from the sweat, which is now evaporating. That is part of it but not all of it. The evidence is at night; even covered up so no evaporation is occurring, the chills linger for minutes. It's cold all the same. The chills are the other side of the coin, the same poor regulation of the body's thermostat going the other way.

There is a two-part action occurring when you place a cold compress on your back. One is that that area is often very hot, and any cooling is good. Two, your heart is there. Cooling the blood going through your heart means it immediately cools whatever part of your body that blood enters.

The thermostat senses the cooler blood, says oh, no need to kick on the cold, so doesn't. Result: hot flash without the ensuing cold chill.

Daytime hot flashes

Minimize the amount of material on your back.

Don't wear blazers or sweaters. If you must wear a blazer or suitcoat, wear a light-weight shirt underneath.

Do not wear camisoles, which put two layers of material right in the spot you need to keep cool, the space between the shoulder blades.

Turn the heat down to 65° F. Wear tops made of thin material.

Before stepping into the car, remove all outer garments like coats, sweaters or jackets, and sit down. Now either place the garment over your front like a blanket, or slide your arms into the coat's arms with the back-of-the-neck tag at your chin. If a hot flash occurs during the commute it's far less dangerous to fling this off than to try to remove a coat while driving. You'll find it keeps you just as warm, if not warmer, than a coat or sweater worn the normal way.

At work or home, if you get cold, put something warm on your lap, a shawl or blanket, instead of a sweater.

The shawl can be a pillowcase, towel, or winter scarf folded double.

A fleece pillowcase is the perfect size for a lap blanket in car or office. These fleece pillowcases are sold at Bed, Bath and Beyond around Christmastime and year around on Amazon.

I bought dark blue fleece pillowcases to match my car's interior; for work, a grey or other subtle color will prevent it from standing out.

To be even more subtle at work, a winter coat scarf, fleece or wool, can be folded and laid on the lap to provide a surprising amount of warmth.

Anything made from cotton will be cold and need warming up.

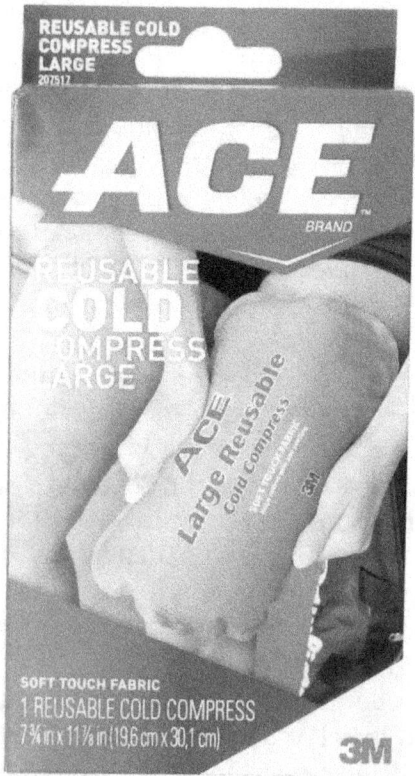

My favorite car and night sweats killer, $11

A fleece throw in the car is fine if you're the passenger, but if you're the driver, use something smaller.

You'll get more hot flashes in the car in winter than summer, due to the coat. Two slippery-skinned refreezeable medical compress(es) can be kept in the door pocket.

Immediately upon getting into the car, slide one cold compress under your collar and then a few inches down to the proper spot on your back. Drive to work normally. It is surprisingly not as uncomfortable as it sounds. Being able to leave your coat on for the whole trip, instead of madly ripping it off in heavy traffic, is priceless.

In winter, simply keep the compresses in the door pocket to chill.

In warm weather, chill in the frig and carry them with you to the car.

A soft-sided square lunchbox chiller can store a few compresses. Left in the car all day, they're still cool for the ride home.

In some cars, not all, the AC routes past the glove compartment, cooling it more than one would think. Check out whether that's the case in your car. If so, stash cold compresses in the glove compartment.

Chilling the source of the hot flash, between the shoulder blades, as quickly as possible is the way to reduce the severity of a hot flash.

If done quickly enough, there's a 20% chance the hot flash can be short circuited completely. Averted.

But not for long. Another will come.

It sometimes it takes a bit of creativity. Some choices:

Move to a different chair.

Move to a different spot in the bed.

Lean against the wall; when that spot heats up, move to a new cool spot.

Cement wall is better than drywall, but both work.

Press your back against a window.

Steel beams are also good to lean against and cool yourself.

Wear a backless dresses. OK, not always good business attire, but I wish it was. It would be great if someone developed a line of clothes for menopause. They would consist of tops with shoulder to wrist fleece arms but just a thin layer over the entire back.

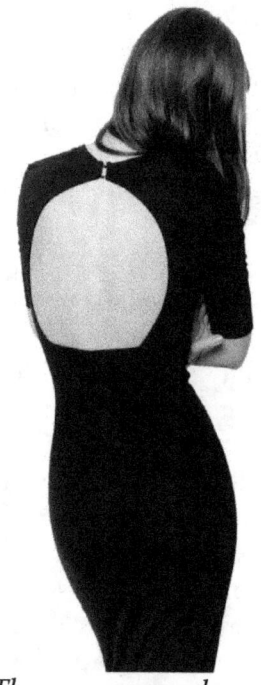

The menopause dress

In winter, step outside. Lean with your back against a wall for immediate chilling.

Cooling your ears or head or whole body help, but aren't as effective as cooling the spine between the shoulder blades.

Cool as much of your body as you can, of course, but if you can apply something cooling to only one part, cool the source. Cooling the head or neck does not prevent the subsequent cold chill.

If you work, chilling your back several times per day without drawing a lot of attention or getting a bunch of questions is necessary.

Juice pouches and juice boxes make wonderful hot flash compresses at work. You can bring several in a briefcase or lunch cooler. If you have a desk, create a lined cooler in one of the drawers for quick silent access to chilled items.

When a hot flash looms, discreetly put one on the source and lean back in your chair. Hold it in place by just leaning back. When the coast is clear, remove it. If someone spots one on your desk, it raises no questions.

Take the warm ones home each night and chill them again.

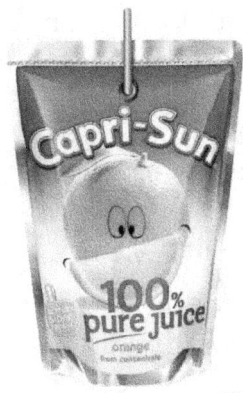

The reusable hot flash cold compress (sans straw)

Keep a few in the department frig for emergencies. Unless you've totally outed yourself as someone in menopause and don't care who knows, don't overdo the juice boxes in the company frig or people will wonder what's up.

The boxes have advantages over pouches. Due to their firm, boxy shape, they are less noisy when handling. Nested tight together they stayed chilled longer, making the last ones much colder by 3 PM than pouches would be. Boxes can be firmly held between back and chair with light pressure. Shifting a bit or rotating them to a cool side doesn't make rustling noises. Using two at a time doubles the area.

Shake or rotate the juice container to gain more coolness out of it.

Drinking: Chugging ice-cold liquid, 10 oz. or more, can minimize a hot flash.

Chills the source from the inside and prevents heat propagation. Use water or calorie-free liquids to prevent sugar buzz or too much caffeine.

Chug the cold liquid quickly, not sips. Drink most of a full bottle if you can. The purpose is to create a decent puddle of cold liquid in your stomach beside the heart, drawing heat away from the inside.

The cold liquid option may be the only one you have during work meetings.

Due to natural body cycles, after 8 PM the house feels miserably cold, even though it's exactly the same temperature it's been all day.

Wearing a sweater backwards is fine when alone or with significant others who are used to your ways, but it's really unacceptable with strangers and acquaintances. The purpose of all this advice is to deal hot flashes but not appear too odd. That purpose is foiled if you're walking around wearing clothes backwards.

Using a lap shawl is just eccentric, not weird. It's not any worse than hiding a little fan heater under the desk. That's my story and I'm sticking to it.

Get some digital thermometers. When the ability to tell whether a room is hot or cold is no longer one of your native powers, external devices are a big help.

These provide temp and humidity, preventing you from annoying others with frequent, "Is it hot in here? Has someone touched the thermostat? Do you feel cold?" Instead of demanding answers from family, nice LED or LCD units are under $10.

~ • ~

Mind control is not the cure to hot flashes. Staving off emotions is not the answer. Living with every minor annoyance or racy joke being highlighted by your own personal clown embarrassing the hell out of you is a terrible burden.

Any strong emotion, even laughter, may set off a hot flash. It might seem if one simply irons out all emotional extremes from one's mental landscape, no more hot flashes.

Today, every single hot flash may come after a strong emotion, but if you succeed in becoming emotionally flat, you'll still get them. They will simply happen every ninety minutes or 200 minutes without any particular emotion.

Despite all your efforts, some hot flashes proceed simply because their time has come.

Night Sweats

These are going to happen no matter what you do. The worst thing is, they're infuriating. At some point, and every night after that, it won't be just the actual hot flash that steams you, it's the anger at the irrationality of it happening AGAIN.

The anger, the boiling "this is so stupid" thoughts, the getting into everything you did wrong that day or some other day or everything someone else did wrong that day . . . all of that keeps you awake for several minutes after the hot flash has gone away.

Step one to dealing with night sweats is counting sheep. Or mediation, or practicing slow breathing and counting off ten veeery slow breaths.

By that I mean you need to find a way to not get irate at night. Even a little is an effective stay-awake tonic.

It's one thing to minimize night sweats once they start, but how much sleep you get at night depends upon how well you recover the bland inattention that sleep requires.

There are a lot of approaches that work to improve falling asleep. One meditation technique that works consists of doing a long, slow exhale to a slow count of four, then inhale on a slow count of four. Count the pairs. Focus on nothing else but lengthening the breathing. Repeat ten times.

The goal is not to get to ten but to nod off prior to reaching ten. Reaching ten can happen if other thoughts intrude. When becoming aware of them, turn them off and continue. It's personal preference whether to continue to ten and start over, start over upon resuming concentration on breathing, or proceed to twenty or more. I continue to ten, then start over.

Many women turn to sleep medications or prescription meds. Those definitely have their place.

Whatever method you use, having night sweats means you will need to get yourself back to sleep several times per night. Your priority is to make your mind bland so you will sleep.

There are many books and articles on sleeping that cover this information using a better bedside manner [pun intended]. If you need help sleeping or returning to sleep, more than meditation, melatonin or over the counter sleep aids can provide, please leave no stone unturned in getting that help, because sleep deprivation makes people cranky and short-tempered. We have enough on our plate without dealing with that.

To handle a night sweat once it's started:

Sleep shirtless. Staving off the onset and quantity of night hot flashes is easier while shirtless. Moving to a cool spot on the bed has a more immediate effect.

If you don't care for sleeping topless, select something that doesn't retain heat on the back. Slippery satin sleepwear seems thin, but the tight weave actually holds in heat quite well. Materials containing small holes, like lace, will work better.

Use only a thin blanket or even just a sheet. Go to the least blanket you can bear.

Wearing warm socks to bed will help make skimpy blanketing bearable. Socks have no effect on night sweat occurrence.

Cold compresses on the back are the quick way to knock out the hot flash at night.

Chill several gel compresses in the frig.

At bedtime, place several under a pillow. Preferably this pillow is beside you, especially for chilling, and not your primary pillow.

If a pillow reserved for keeping compresses cold isn't possible, then a few under your primary pillow is better than nothing. Your head may warm them quicker, but they'll still be cold at 3 AM.

When a hot flash wakes you, pull out a cold compress and lay on it. You might doze off, good.

If it fully warms before the hot flash is gone, pull out another and put the spent one on the floor.

It isn't mandatory to remove the used ones, but leaving the fish-like things in the bed may be distracting when bumped into several hours later.

Moving to a new (cool) spot on the bed in conjunction with the cold compress is even better.

There are hot flash pillows and chillows and flat pillow-cools on the market. Search Amazon under "Health and Personal Care" for "cool pads."

These are all good. Just be aware that one will not last the whole night. If you lay on one cool anything, two hours later that puppy will almost burn your hand. It gets stunningly hot. You'll need three to five of them to get through the night during the worst of the night sweats.

Beware !! You may want to freeze them, and then sleep shirtless, so without thinking you put the freezer-cold item directly on bare skin.

Don't put freezer-chilled compresses directly on bare skin. This will cause freezer burn on your skin. Even worse, it can cause deep tissue damage. You want to chill your blood but not kill skin cells or worse. This is like smoking in bed. You may think you won't nod off, you'll be aware enough to catch it if the pure cold and not moving and forty pounds of pressure holding an ice cube to your skin is causing damage, but you won't.

Sleeves out of flour sack dish towels, pillowcases, cloth bag shoes come in, really anything can be used to put a layer of material between you and an ice-cold compress.

As menopause proceeds, you'll find that it no longer takes freezer-chilled compresses to do the trick against your heat-generating furnace, refrigerated ones work fine. In time, you'll find that gel compresses simply left on the nightstand at room temperature, which is probably 65° F, suffice. Then, in even more time, simply moving to a cool spot in the bed or laying on your side while exposing your bare back to the air is all it takes.

Special Situations

Don't be so quick to cease birth control methods when you enter menopause. You can get pregnant if one of those intermittent menstrual periods is sneaking up on you.

Getting pregnant at a late age is easier to do if you have been pregnant before. To generalize, it's easier for a 45 year old woman to conceive a child if this would be her fourth child than if it's her first. The reason could be that nature's ancient blunt tool, genetics, deals only with statistical likelihoods and not specifics. It's statistically more likely a woman who has other children has a support network in place to bring this one to adulthood. A woman who for whatever reason (genetics has no notion of birth control) hasn't been pregnant by 45 is probably going to have trouble raising it.

Another way of viewing it is that nature plays along. If a woman, for whatever reason, isn't pregnant by 45, it's probably because that's her intention. Nature doesn't dive down into the details, it's kind of a broad generalities tool. The longer a woman has never gotten pregnant, the more the body closes up shop, doesn't keep things set up for the arrival of a little package.

Often women and their doctors jump too soon to that advantage of menopause, being able to cease using birth control. Many late-age pregnancies resulted from this.

Take your pregnancy precautions through the first two years. Once your periods are irregular, there is no telling when it's safe and when it's not.

It's hardly going to be a big comfort to know that a high percentage of these pregnancies end in miscarriage. To a lot of women, that is worse than having a baby. It absolutely would be the case for me. Having a late-age pregnancy turn into a miscarriage is not the good news; it's the life-changing-news-turned-into-devastating news.

But not everyone is like me. Some people, for medical or other reasons, just can't harbor a pregnancy or undergo childbirth right now. So for the first time in their lives they have to deal with making a decision that any other time in their lives would be unthinkable. They damn their own weakness, their body, their situation. Some even feel it would be better to die than terminate. When someone says the risk is 20% and another puts it at 40%, what does that mean? When it's important health-related or personal situation conditions, 20%, 40%, it is all meaningless because your case is one bite at the apple. How your actual one turns out is what it ends up being. It doesn't matter how correct and right anyone was when they assigned your risk to be 5%. If you end up being in that 5%, it's 100% to you.

The woman and her husband might feel they'll die of shame if she makes the sensible decision. How will their other children feel? Other children . . . sob.

This is deep serious stuff, these late-age pregnancies. It's so much better to never cross that bridge. Don't consider yourself out of range until it's been more than fourteen months since your last period.

How many doctors tell you to expect your period to return now and then for up to three years after your first struggles with hot flashes? Mine didn't. Menopause can have intermittent remission over a two-year span.

Because no hint of this was ever shared with me by doctors or the menopause books and pamphlets I read, I gave my leftover tampons and napkins away to a teenager. Then two months later I had to buy more. Four months later I gave those away too. Then I had to buy more again. By then, genius that I am, I saw a pattern. I didn't give them away any more. Good thing too, because I needed them again.

Menopause isn't a fall from a cliff. There is no start date and end date. Most of us have a view of the start only in the rear view mirror. The start of menopause ramps up. One day the symptoms increase to the point where a woman says, yep, this is definitely a hot flash—but in my case I wasn't the one. I described the sensation to a friend who laughed and told ME it's a hot flash. Even that day could not be called the start, because it began long before that.

How far back did it go? What about being really hot in the car during the drive to work these past two months, were those hot flashes? What about that quarrel I had three months ago that the bedroom was too hot, we're wasting energy keeping it this warm only to sleep without covers—was that a night sweat?

Being hot, taking off a sweater, feeling like hitting the pool, all of those are normal occurrences so do not set off any alarm bells that menopause is starting.

What about using your period as a way to set the menopause 'start month?' If you are in menopause, you already know the answer. That didn't stop on a dime either. Getting irregular is a symptom, but we've all had that before so all by itself it means nothing.

The month menopause started is as hard to pin down as the day a child was potty-trained. When my son was small, acquaintances would ask "Is he potty-trained yet?" My answer was: "No one is ever fully potty-trained; we just go longer and longer between accidents."

Menopause is like that too. At some point you know you are really in the middle of it. But when did it start? Narrowing it down to first half or last half of a certain year may be the closest you can get, and if your life was busy so you weren't being observant, picking a year may be the best you can do. Don't feel bad about this. If your doctor is clueless enough to think any woman can provide a real start month, almost everything he or she says about menopause after that is suspect.

Don't give away or throw way your menstrual stuff for at least two years after your last period. Heck, hang onto all of it anyway, in case visitors or guests need them. I store mine in the cabinet in the guest bathroom. That's always a nice thing to do, especially if your visitors are teenage girls or young women. They're new at this and are bad at estimating how many they'll need for the day or when they'll need them.

Travel

Travel throws a wrench into the works of menopause. It actually throws a wrench into the menstrual cycle of many women who travel. The timing of your period may change when sleeping away from home.

To explain why this is so, it will require a bit of background on biology and believe it or not, anthropology.

Going back fifty generations and even 500 generations, humans lived in small groups of related individuals. We paired up, and men were responsible for their offspring with their mate. While women can be certain the baby is theirs, all that engenders that same confidence in men is knowing they were present at the conception.

Back then, men would go off in hunting parties, the entire group of adult males in a tribe either being there or being away concurrently. How would a man know if someone else from some other tribe had lain with his wife while he was gone? Well, he wouldn't know. But it makes genetic sense to improve the odds that the pair-bonded male who expends a great deal of energy providing for and raising offspring has a reason to feel they are all his own.

Nature had a system in place to do exactly that. It was a pretty good system. It gave every father almost rock-solid certainty that the child born is his—or know with almost no doubt that it was not his. Fifty generations is an eyeblink in genetic terms, so that system is still in place. But as we all know, it doesn't work anymore in modern society. The residual effect that we see today is just an annoyance to high school girls and to women who travel.

What worked fine in small hunter-gatherer tribes does not work in cities, does not work in offices, factories, or suburbs.

Here's what's going on:

When women live together, their periods align. This is a biological reality. While there has never been any secret about it in science or folk wisdom, neither has it been assigned any particular value or significance. It falls into the realm of trivia.

Being raised in a household with three daughters a bit over a year apart, I first noticed it when I was about fifteen and month after month our box of Kotex®, which sat there full for three weeks, was emptied in two days.

My major in college was archeology with a strong side of anthropology, and I don't recall this minor biological imperative ever playing a part in anyone's theory of early man. Surprisingly, it's actually key to human history.

Something as profound as women's reproductive cycles having a never-fail synchronization policy cannot be just a pointless biological accident. It's the reason why tribe-sized social groupings could function at all in a species whose sex drive is always 'on.'

Most species have seasonal estrus cycles, and males biologically develop interest when notified by a scent produced by females, or by time of year. When it is not the season, neither sex has any particular sex drive. Sure, there can be dominance and territorial fighting, but these are related to survival, which is only indirectly linked to reproduction and even less to physical sex itself. Most species are very clear on the purpose for sex, and it's not for pleasure. For many species it's deadly business, as in competitors may die. But when the switch is off, it's off.

When human women spend time together, an alpha or primary female pulls the cycle of the other females into alignment with hers via scent. None of the women are aware this is happening, or who is alpha. The means by which this happens is usually by speeding up the onset of by several days, but it can also be done by lengthening it a few days. It doesn't happen every time with every long bus ride or overnight stay in a hotel bed slept on by a different woman the night before, because that other woman might not be more 'alpha.'

The studies of this are pretty meager, but what constitutes an 'alpha' female as far as period timing goes may have little to do with social dominance. It goes without saying if the group of women are ruled by a post-menopausal woman, that woman has no effect at all on their cycles.

What was the useful function of this in tribal times? All the women in the group became fertile in the same few days every month. Because men require several hours between sex acts, this meant that one man could never father all the children in a tribe, even if he was a big bully. A man who performs the act a handful of hours later will have an ejaculation relatively devoid of sperm. But never mind that. Concurrent periods means concurrent fertility therefore concurrent pregnancies. On a schedule that pretty much matched the moon. Even if the men traveled far and wide hunting, it wasn't rocket science to plan to be home during the fertility week.

This concurrent pregnancy imperative worked to everyone's benefit; women had nursing backup and the children had age mates to play with.

Since nursing moms might go 18 months between births, age group lumps were created in the tribe. Kids like age group lumps. They are hard-wired to be easier to teach in age group lumps. That's why two kids are such a handful and 25 kids are manageable by one person. That's why a single adult can get 25 kids to stick to a task for hours while trying to get one kid alone to do the same is a never-ending battle.

If one kid takes X amount of energy to control and amuse, it ought to take 25X to do the same with 25, but it does not. It takes about 1.5X. That's because kids are hard-wired to function that way. The reason humans evolved the way we did, why we can have schools where hundreds of kids obey two dozen adults for hours on end is because when women hang together a few hours a day, their fertility cycles align.

If a three-day fertility window passed while the men were gone, no one should be pregnant. There should be a month of no pregnancies. The whole tribe would instantly know if a pregnancy happened while the men were out of town, because the fertility week was as common knowledge as observing the phase of the moon.

Since all the adult women knew the fertility week, even if they dallied with other men, it was possible to ensure all their offspring were their husband's.

What does all that mean to you? It means when you start a new job or sleep in hotels or stay with relatives, your period cycle may get messed up. Not always, and if you happen to have an alpha cycle, perhaps you will never experience it. If you're middle of the pack, not alpha and not lowest, you'll see it only occasionally. If your cycle is very far from alpha, you will have irregular periods your whole life, because every day-long conference, day-long tour, and hotel bed will pull your cycle one way or another.

What does this have to do with menopause? For the first two years of menopause, travel can jump-start your period again. So pack a few tampons, or even enough for a full period if you will be staying in hotels or in a home containing younger females.

Many menopausal women report the same experience. Their story sounds like this: "can you believe it? We went to Florida and I thought great, for the first time I don't have to pack a bunch of tampons because I haven't had a period for nine months, and I'm there only three days and it starts."

Bring your supplies when you're going on vacation, staying in a hotel or with other people, even if it's been over a year since your last period. When it happened to me quite a long time after hot flashes started, I felt . . . flattered. Hello, old friend. One last time. I'm not so over the hill. It felt like an old boyfriend buying me a drink. We have different lives now, but for a bit I am young again. Still a sexy creature.

Food and Menopause

There are a lot of books touting different diets to reduce menopause symptoms. If they work at all it is due to the placebo effect. So give it a shot; if it works for you, wonderful.

There's evidence that fat cells generate low levels of estrogen, so it may be the case that heavier people have milder hot flashes than thin people. Milder does not mean pleasant or not annoying. It's such a relative term, and people really know only their personal case, so who can be certain more weight means milder symptoms for any one person?

Changing your diet for menopause makes you feel like you're doing something constructive. The urge to do something can be overpowering. If that helps you and doesn't lead to imbalances, go for it.

In the throes of the worst of your hot flashes, using diet, vitamins or exercise to quell symptoms is like putting your hand out when a car is coming at you at 30 MPH. It doesn't stop the car from hitting you, but you still very much want to put out your hand.

It's a different story three or five years later. When the symptoms are milder due to the natural passage of time, taking a daily vitamin seems to reduce the severity of night sweats that particular night. If it reduces even one of them just enough to prevent waking, that's fifteen minutes more sleep. Those minutes add up.

Exercise may reduce the severity of night sweats—for the evening of the day you exercised. It's a daily thing, works for one day. It won't amount to a perceptible improvement when still in the drenched-with-sweat stages, but when hot flashes are down to merely uncomfortably warm, thirty minutes of brisk walking or heaving around eight-pound free weights for twenty minutes while watching TV can make a 50% difference in nighttime severity. Eight years after my first hot flash, exercise anytime during the day makes the difference between waking up three times to move to a new spot in the bed due to heat, or only doing it once. Vitamin plus exercise works even better.

One word about vitamins: get the kind that do not have 18 mg. of iron. That could be any of the ones targeted at men, children or older women. The idea behind that much iron is to compensate for monthly iron loss.

If you have half of a huge bottle left, don't throw them out; simply buy another kind with smaller amounts or no iron and take the ones with iron only two or three times per week until the bottle is gone. Excess iron can cause other problems, but you'd need to have far more than typical vitamin iron levels to see those.

In case you don't keep up with nutritional news, the jury is in on the cause of the drastic increase in diabetes: twenty years of cutting fat from our diets. This is a long story based on copious research, and I encourage you to read what Consumer Reports has to say on it. To be so brief that it risks being misunderstood, when people reduced fat in their diets, they increased sugar and starchy food. These require a spike in insulin to digest, and over the years causes pancreas fatigue. When people 'kick' diabetes by losing 40 pounds, or even as little as 20 pounds, what happens is they are giving their pancreas a rest and it heals.

Not all calories are equal; a nice juicy Italian sausage or bratwurst can put less into fat cells than an unrelenting low fat, high starch, high sugar diet.

There's another aspect of weight gain that keeps a low profile. Nutritionists probably think knowing it can't lead to good choices, but I find that paternalistic.

Let's call it the "Thanksgiving Dinner phenomenon" because it doesn't have a name. If you want the scientific details and not the analogy version of the biology, it's well documented.

Our bodies adapt to our usual diet. Food digestion is actually stunningly complex. It involves molecule breakdown, sorting out the nutrients, the vitamins, the useful metals into teeny tiny bits and phasing them into the blood stream. Triage, mix, match, convert, count . . . it's like 4,000 little men working at full steam, doing hundreds of things each minute, every time we eat a meal. There are a thousand little blood vessels and several organs picking out the parts they need, doing their process to them, and distributing them to the blood stream in timed-release amounts, or putting them into storage, whichever their operating instructions guide them to do.

This functions fine when a person eats a nice little 700 calorie meal, or even a bag of microwave popcorn with extra butter, or even a big piece of cheesecake. But what if all three are done within 45 minutes? The 4,000 little men get overwhelmed. Like Lucille Ball on the candy assembly line, it's all coming too fast. No, they don't eat it like she did, they let it go by. They work only so fast, and anything more just gets past them untouched.

This means that a Thanksgiving dinner doesn't pack on as much weight as you think it would.

Scientists have come up with a number. It probably varies for everyone.

The number is . . . 2,500 calories. If you eat more than 2,500 calories at one sitting, the calories over 2,500 are going to flow through untouched. As if they were never consumed. Your system simply tops out.

Now, 2,500 calories in one sitting is a lot of food, more than you need all day. But if you've exceeded that already and your sister says 'just try a sliver of the pecan pie' you might as well. You can't use the excuse that it will put on weight.

Roughage: Roughage helps move food through the system, reducing the contact with your 4,000 little men, possibly allowing maybe 80 calories from a 1,000 calorie meal to flow by ungrabbed. Again, dangerous information that you must promise you won't abuse: there are people who abuse laxatives for this very reason. They take more than the recommended amount more often than manufacturer's instructions state, to rush the food through their system to reduce calorie absorption.

Taking a laxative now and then, say once every two weeks, for whatever reason you find meaningful, is the intended use of the product. Taking them more often can cause a dependence, and a lot of trouble when you try to stop, so don't do that.

Roughage tabs are perfect for moving food at a good pace through the system. Roughage products like Fiber Choice®, Metamucil® and others can be taken every day all year long and do only good for your system.

Roughage is good for daily use, laxatives once or twice a month tops. Follow a big meal with a couple of chewable fiber tablets or other source of roughage. That's exactly when they are most effective, with a meal.

If you take too many roughage tablets or roughage gummies, it will have an opposite effect, not producing loose and easy stools. Too much roughage, such as four or five times the daily recommended amount will create hard and stubborn bowel movements. Simply correct the dosage tomorrow. No harm, no foul.

It's good to have what are called loose, unstraining stools; if you're straining to poo, and the poo is more solid and round-ballish, it means the food producing that poo stayed in your intestines several hours longer. Every possible nutrient and calorie was wrung out of it in those hours. The little men can work on only the food passing right before them, and the slower it moves, the more time they have to pick through. If it's moving faster, they have time to grab only the key stuff, then it's out of reach.

Your body has very good operating instructions: if you're low on say, Vitamin B, your little men are going to reach for the Vitamin B first. Have no worries on that regard, you'll get the nutrients you need from your food when roughage is moving it through at a smooth clip. The roughage speed is the speed the human gut was designed to take.

When you use laxatives, not so much. It's going way too fast. You can get vitamin deficiencies from taking laxatives too often even if you take a vitamin pill. With laxatives that vitamin pill will still be half a lump when coming out the other end.

Weight Gain

There are three parts to losing or maintaining weight: fighting the hungries, changing the habitual serving size or frequency, and moving around more.

It's nice if you do all three, but dieting to lose weight can be successful with any two. To merely stop gaining weight or lose a few pounds per year, do one of them.

Serving Size

Changing the habitual serving size and frequency may need to be done on only a handful of commonly eaten foods.

It's plausible some foods can be exempt from portion size change. Say, a twice-a-year hot fudge sundae. Or a baked potato.

Even with exemptions, weight loss will not last unless you ratchet down your mental picture of serving size and frequency. Exercise as a weight loss method works well, but no one keeps it up forever. Unless your day job is bike messenger or construction worker, exercise is optional extra work you make for yourself.

Modifying the idea of a portion, making it your new habit, is an easy way to counteract the glacier-like force of menopause weight gain.

Years ago, in my mind a serving of cereal or oatmeal was in a certain-size bowl, filled to the brim. Today, another, much smaller bowl filled with cereal and milk only to a point a half inch below the brim is a serving. It took years.

A candy bar used to be my idea of a serving of chocolate; now a little puddle of M&Ms® or four mini-eggs (I stock up at Easter), about 1/3 of a candy bar in volume, is a serving size. Changing portion size took time and attention, but once done, it feels natural. Eating is still on auto-pilot.

A yogurt with granola used to feel like half a breakfast; now it suffices for the whole breakfast. I would weigh more today if I hadn't adjusted my idea of serving size.

Nature helps with this process. A tummy distended by eating too much is more painful at 55 than it was at 25. Reflux, indigestion, and trouble sleeping at night are the come-along buddies of huge meals. An overactive reflux condition can provide motivation to skip late-night snacking and drinking before bed.

Most people start to cut back on serving size naturally, without effort, as they grow older. Unfortunately, the size of our dishes and the way we shop and prepare food foils this natural tendency. Who wants to waste food? Ceasing to eat when there are four bites left on the plate is often hard to do. It's absolutely what should be done; we know that, but some deeper voice is telling us to finish up. Probably mom's.

Sometimes all you need to do is go with your gut. Let your gut rule. Do not finish that ice cream cone if the interest is gone. Don't eat that last chicken wing merely to remove the need to put it in a plastic bag in the frig.

Find a way to make it OK, in your mind, to drop the last few mouthfuls on the plate into the garbage can. Make it OK to feed the garbage can so you skip the last 150 calories of the meal. Think of it like a pet you feed. In fact, a dog probably works far better. I'll bet that's why people who own dogs are statistically thinner; it isn't the dog walking, it's the last four bites on the plate, day after day.

~ • ~

As an aside, to those who have a dog and feel giving them a portion of your meal encourages begging, the appropriate way to do it is to always feed the dog from his dish. People food is no different than what is contained in dog food; dog food is simply blended and food colored to match our idea of dog food, with some added bits like bones and innards that don't appeal to our sensibilities but are necessary parts of a dog's menu. If your dog consistently gets meals in a certain location, he will eventually sit by his dish at mealtimes.

~ • ~

The French have a custom of feeding you until you can't eat anymore, meaning some food is on your plate and you won't eat it.

Americans visiting France wonder why they are pestered to take a dessert after finishing dinner, and the host won't take no for an answer. The reason is because the Americans cleaned their plate. They would need to leave two good morsels on the plate for the server to believe they were full.

We should all be like that.

Re-learn to leave something on the plate. Theoretically, it's implausible a restaurant serves us exactly the amount of food that fills us up, not one mouthful too much or too little.

Food comes in portions: one piece of chicken or two, a hard-boiled egg, a piece of cake. Our actual satiation is probably at 1.75 pieces of chicken, or even 1.3 pieces. We force down the rest out of obligation.

Obligation to who? To what? That is the question. Reach deep down inside to answer that question for yourself.

Diet food: Many companies thrive by convincing Americans that diet food is specially purchased food. Not regular food. You pay for expensive processed meals while dieting, and stop when you are done.

While I concede this may be necessary for the very obese, and it works splendidly for adjusting mental portion size (thank you, Lean Cuisine®!), it's very unsustainability makes it unviable for a life strategy of fitting into airline seats without needing a seatbelt extender.

Well, now I'm going to backpedal. If you allow your diet and habits to flip entirely, the diet food becoming the normal diet, it works. This assumes the diet food is available in the grocery store. I eat Lean Cuisines for lunch almost every work day because they taste good and I like them. Since 2001.

The half-a-grapefruit, celery as veggie, steak-without-potato-or-bread diets have little chance of morphing into your normal daily lifestyle. Vegetables without butter at every meal and always pulling the skin off chicken as a way of life, oh shoot me now.

There is a lot to be said for the dinky portion diet. When you dine out with friends or family, perhaps you get by with a taste from their plates. It's possible to have a 400 calorie dinner with a few forkfuls placed on your bread plate plus a bread. When dining with kids, it's a breeze to get their whole veggie serving; add a drink and it's a diet meal.

Diets that prevent you from eating at restaurants with friends and family are not any good. They are worse than useless; they can harm the most important part of your life, your connections with friends and family.

I have refused dinner invitations, restaurant meetings, and day-long excursions simply because of dieting, and frankly, I think I would have more friends today if I hadn't said no.

Besides, it often happens that one can feel full after finishing the salad and two rolls. In the past you may have plowed on and ate the whole meal anyway. Instead of treating the actual shove-food-in-mouth part as the sociable part, consider that just being there and talking is the sociable part. A month later your fellow diners may quote you or tell others what fun you all had that day, but they have forgotten what you ate.

Honor your gut when the salad has pretty much filled you up; nibble down the parts of your meal that don't reheat well, and take home the rest for tomorrow.

Fighting the Hungries

Diet pills and chewies are great. Quite a few of them can make you feel less hungry, which is good, but you still have to eat less.

If you feel less hungry but don't reduce portion size or frequency, the appetite suppressant will not help much.

For most of us, just reducing portion size of snacks, plus eating at meals until the edge of hunger is gone— and no more—will stop weight gain or slow it to a glacier pace. It won't cause the weight to peel off. Appetite suppressants can help you get to the next level, enable you to consume fewer calories than you burn off, day after day.

There are three basic kinds: one, those with appetite suppressants and metabolism boosters, mainly caffeine and other energizers, that make it easier to become active.

Two, the kind that work best when combined with exercise; they don't do much when weight-bearing exercise isn't performed regularly. Those who combine them with exercise are very impressed.

Three, the kind that suppress appetite without any energizer component. The third kind is best for fighting after-dinner and late evening urges to snack.

Not eating after 7 PM is a big step towards losing weight. Not only will you eat fewer calories that particular day, but the next morning most people will find they aren't appreciably more hungry.

Hydroxycut® Gummies fall into the third category. They are effective in quelling the distracting hungry urge. Taking two can diminish the late afternoon urge to snack. In the evenings it's pretty hard to resist the lure of that can of cashews or ice cream. Savoring two Gummies provides resistance strength. Their effect lasts about 90 minutes. While the pair of gummies contain thirty calories, each time I take them they save me from eating 250.

For coffee drinkers who get enough caffeine already, those who want to limit their caffeine intake, or those who find the hardest part of sticking to a diet is shortly before bed, the Gummies and other non-energizing types are best.

Of course, taking two gummies and then stopping at a Taco Bell will have no effect. I'll still order what I always order because that's my habit. Taco Bell doesn't sell half a burrito.

~ • ~

There are medical solutions for enforcing a reduced portion diet, stomach stapling and the like. If you are contemplating that, your doctor and websites devoted to that topic are appropriate places for getting information.

This chapter speaks mainly to women who up until now were a normal weight, or were OK with their weight, and are now getting less happy with it.

It may be out of step with most menopause books to be all for appetite suppressants. I was all for painkillers during childbirth too.

The point is often made that the weight comes back on after losing a decent amount by using appetite suppressants. That is meaningless. Rather, it only has meaning if you compare two completely different individuals. When you stick to talking about one person, some weight loss is always better than no weight loss.

Here's why.

Example: A 53 year old woman who weighs 170 lbs. starts dieting on her birthday with the help of appetite suppressants. She takes them, along with portion size and exercise changes, for 6 months.

When she turns 54, she weighs 152.

When she turns 55, she weighs 160.

When she turns 56, she weighs 170.

In this light, if she hadn't had the help of appetite suppressants, what would she weigh at 56?

Not 170, that's for certain. Victory!

At 56 she weighs exactly what she weighed at 53.

What if she used them again and turned 60 weighing the same as 53? Wonderful!

~ • ~

Losing weight doesn't have to be more painful than necessary. Just like childbirth. The child is born just the same if it doesn't hurt much. With appetite suppressants like Hydroxycut Gummies, the weight is gone even if you weren't crazy, obsessively hungry for six hours a day.

If appetite suppressants make your day, even this one hour, less miserable, I'm all for it. The goal you are working towards is turning the weight clock back to a weight you used to be. At our age, we're not aiming for a modeling career. We just want to use our nice clothes for another few years.

Ratcheting back your weight a year or two every few years is wonderful, and enough. It reduces your chances of diabetes, or if you have it, can improve it enough to move off injectable medication.

Less weight is easier on the joints. It means you have a bigger wardrobe because everything you've purchased in the past 8 years fits [more or less]. Anyone who tries to tell you this isn't good enough is full of baloney. It's absolutely perfect.

If you glance at stories on the internet about appetite suppressants, you might get the impression they are dangerous. There is a lot of fabricating and exaggerating on both sides of the fence. Those who sell appetite suppressants and those who oppose them all make extreme claims.

Consumer Reports, not known for sugar-coating a bad product, acknowledges there are several appetite suppressants on the market that suppress appetite with negligible side effects. Their view, similar to mine, is that it takes individual trial and error to find a good fit.

To find a product that works for you, visit the drugstore, read labels, and give a few things a shot. As is the case with antacids; each one works GREAT for 25%, OK for another 40%, and are meh or make things worse for the rest. If you don't like the buzz or it makes you queasy, try another. Don't keep taking it unless you think you can learn to live with the side effect.

This is one medication where the excuse, "it made me light-headed, probably because I took it on an empty stomach" can't be used. The idea is that it will always be taken on an empty stomach, that's the point. If you can't abide the feeling when you take it on an empty stomach, try something else.

~ • ~

Diet-assisting potions aren't cheap. Before you dismiss trying them due to the price, consider that you may actually save money. If it works, the savings will be in fewer snack foods and making three meals out of the ingredients that used to produce two.

A restaurant meal you used to chow down in one sitting now produces a doggy bag that becomes supper tomorrow, a two-fer. The appetite suppressants may cost $50 a month but save $70 on the food bill.

When weight gain is viewed over time, all phases where you ratchet-back to a lower weight are a good thing. EVERYBODY weighs more at 60 than they did at 18, unless they're sick.

The question is, how much more. If I ratchet my weight back to my 38-year-old weight four times in fifteen years, so I reach 60 weighing only six pounds more than I did at 38, give me a gold star!

That's my story and I'm sticking to it.

~ • ~

What about those stories about kidney failure and other bad things caused by appetite suppressants?

In every case the person involved had overdosed. Not just accidentally taken them twice in a day a few times, but was deliberately taking six to twenty times the recommended dosage frequently, or was taking more than five times the recommended dosage for months. Some cases involved taking it with drugs specifically contraindicated on the label.

Follow the label instructions. Stick to the bottle dosage, don't nudge over the recommended amount more than one day out of seven, look at the drug conflicts and make sure you absolutely are not taking any of those and you'll be fine.

Ephedra, a wonderful appetite suppressant and one I used to lose forty pounds [and kept it off for twelve years], was removed from the market in the early 2000s due to nutcases who took handfuls of pills at a time. Their organ failure and even death, however, is no different than would happen with that level of overdose involving many over-the-counter medications, such as allergy, pain killers, and flu treatments. Even some of the spices in your spice rack would cause organ failure in large doses.

Many OTC medications are harmful at high doses. Even drinking twenty cups of coffee at once will land you in the hospital. No one suggests banning coffee because some fool might slug down twenty espressos.

Why they singled out this one very effective drug for removal from the market is troubling. The current standard for OTC treatments does not require them to be perfectly safe at ten times the recommended dosage. It is a slippery slope to ban a drug for failure to be safe at overdose levels, because almost none of our ordinary medications or treatments could pass that test.

I'm not getting on any bandwagons to bring back OTC Ephedra, but it should be allowed again. It's fine if it finds a place beside codeine-containing cough medicines, behind the pharmacy counter and available only upon asking the Pharmacist, but it doesn't deserve being banned.

Moving Around

Encouraging exercise is fine, but it is not always an option for every woman who needs to lose weight. We risk aggravating joint injuries, are more prone to tendon injuries, and even cuts and bruises take longer to heal than they once did.

Sometimes losing weight must be done without a significant increase in exercise, or rather 'exercise' as defined by the exercise industry. Let's put aside the definition propagated by the money-making proponents of exercise and open it up to include moving around, or exercise not requiring special shoes or memberships.

The opposite of exercise is being non-energetic and sitting still on the couch. In this light, all motion is worthwhile and counts as exercise.

~ • ~

There was a study years ago with Navajo Indians as the subjects and middle-age weight gain as the issue. The subjects were on a controlled diet and exercise regimen, yet the researchers were having trouble making sense of their numbers and results.

Then someone sorted their study group into high-fidgeters and low fidgeters, and voila! Perfect sense. High fidgeters wore off 200 calories more per day than the lowest fidgeters.

Don't sniff at that; it amounts to half a pound per week, or over twenty pounds per year. Unlike getting-sweaty exercise plans, a natural fidgeter doesn't take a day off. The shifting and foot-tapping and arm movements can continue every waking hour.

As Richard Simmons says, just get moving! All movement is good. Dance a little while stirring food on the stove, do the YMCA arm movements while sitting on the toilet. Do leg lifts while reading a book. It sounds funny, but integrating more movement into your daily life in a manner that doesn't embarrass you or cause questions is the way to go.

Movement begets movement. If you start modestly with any increase, from going up and down the stairs a few times more per day or parking in the farthest-away parking spot you can find, in just a few weeks it gets easier. Sore muscles never have to happen. It doesn't have to be 'no pain, no gain;' you can just work up slowly.

Every time you move around, it becomes slightly easier to do it again two days from now. Try lifting a bag of flour over your head ten times before opening it. Integrate small additional motions into normal tasks. Just by moving more the movement becomes easier, so in the future you do it even more, with less effort. When it's less hard to do, the effort isn't an impediment. If you decide to walk up and down a staircase several times, don't forget to use your arms to pull yourself up. It's all good.

Once I used to do five mile runs ten times a year. Jogging is no longer a good option for me because it will lead to knee problems and shin splints.

The type of walking machine called an elliptical provides both arm and leg exercise. Most of them are quieter than treadmills, making it easier to watch TV or movies while working out. They allow a pace and effort that is even lighter than plain walking. It's all good.

A few exercise tips: Two gallon milk jugs filled with water make good free weights. If you really get into it you might want to buy some, but you don't need to spend money to 'do it right.' It's all good.

Do push-ups with your hands on a table, countertop, or armrest of the couch. When you get up to 25, try a lower surface. Or just go for fifty on the same piece of furniture. When you start, you may manage to do only two deep ones. Do several little half or even ¼ pushups after you no longer can do full ones. Adding these at the end accelerate the process of getting to 25.

That's true of all lifting exercises; do little shortie 2" or 5" ones after you no longer can do full ones. Making a rule to stop doing pushups, situps or other lifting or pushing once a full one can no longer be done means it will take twice as long to get to 25. The little shortie ones are the key to getting stronger fast.

Another key is to take rests and resume. When the muscles start to burn a bit, pause. A fifteen second rest between tries allows you do to a few more today. That's what really matters: how many you do today.

There is no rule they have to be all in a row. Take a two minute break or even five minute break and pick up the count where you left off. If you can do forty today over the span of an hour, that's a heck of a lot better than doing six, struggling on the seventh so calling it quits. The body progresses based on forty.

Not only that, if twenty-five of those are half-lifts, the body counts that as twelve. It's all good.

Do what the professional body builders and athletes do: push yourself every other day, or even every third day.

If the muscles feel a little sore the next day, skip it. If they are fine, go ahead.

Giving the muscles a rest is not indulgent; it's how getting strong works. Muscles grow, believe it or not, by developing little tears that heal with more muscle in the gaps. The soreness means growing.

Muscle mass is a good thing; a square inch of muscle weighs seven times more than a square inch of fat. More than that, muscle has a higher energy demand just to be fed and hang around. If you weigh 180 pounds but have ten pounds more muscle on you than another 180 pound person, you can eat more and not gain weight.

After the Olympics, gold-medal swimmer Michael Phelps submitted to a study which showed he burned about 280 calories per hour just sitting down watching TV. Sigh.

What if you don't rest between sore-muscle-creating exercise, but work though it? You may become strong but wiry. You've heard the saying, right? It means someone who is stronger than he looks, strong but skinny-looking. Usually used in reference to a guy who didn't grow muscle mass because he got up and did the same work as yesterday, even though he was hurting. That may be fine if you're a jockey or chimney sweep, but most of us want muscle-looking muscles and the resulting metabolism boost.

Another thing the pros do is split the body, working legs one day and arms the next. This way they go to the gym every day yet still give the muscles the rest they need. If you're sore all over, give it a day. But if your legs are sore, do some arm things, and vice versa. It's all good.

I'm not being specific about actual movements and exercises because there are so many books that cover this. Every proponent thinks their type is perfect, but it boils down to what you want to do. Yoga, tai chi, pole dancing, Jazzercize, pilates, cycling, rowing, tae kwon do, karate, elliptical, jogging, swimming laps, rock climbing, golf, buckets of balls at the driving range, stairmaster, free weights, weight-lifting, spinning, and belly dancing are some of them.

YMCA and community centers have weekly or bi-weekly fitness classes too. If you try one of these, don't be discouraged upon seeing the others. Some people have done it for years and it's your first month, so you have a way to go before you look like that. Remind yourself that the good ones had a day like your day today, being the worst in the class. Or pretty close to it. They shook it off and kept attending. All motion is good.

Just dancing around the house is sufficient exercise. "Dancing' means moving around to music, no judgment. It means butt-wiggling or knee lifting while doing something else. My experience is, if you start dancing to the radio, favorite songs or even TV commercial jingles, or just sing a song and dance to that, and keep doing it for a few weeks, your motions will get steadier and stronger. You'll never have to make a forced march out of exercising, just waltz around the living room. All motion is good.

If you want something more strenuous for low cost, consider jumping rope. This needs a bit more ceiling height than most homes have, but it might work for you. It's great for an apartment with a little deck. If you are planning to start jogging, this is a great way to strengthen your ankles and calf muscles and ramp up your lung capacity before going public. If anything goes amiss, at least you are not ten blocks from home.

Start with the skipping style, one foot then the other. Play around with which foot is in front. Mix it up.

The rope can be anything; old clothes line works the best. Regular jump ropes with handles are frequently sold at rummage sales.

When starting leg exercises, or even the day after a lot of walking, your legs may cramp up that night.

In the morning, before you get out of bed:

1) massage your calf muscles;

2) stretch your Achilles tendon by pulling your toes up towards your knee.

If your bed has a footboard, you can use that to stretch your feet. Another thing that may work to prevent or reduce leg cramps is taking Omega-3 fish oil, three 1000 mg. capsules, with a meal or snack.

Like any treatment, fish oil may not work 100% of the time for everyone. The stretching and massaging, though, will always be a big help.

There are other causes of night leg cramps, but this refers only to the ones caused by ramping up the exercise level.

Some people benefit the most when they have an exercise buddy. Someone they walk with at lunch every day, or meet at the gym on agreed-upon days. Someone they jog with in the park or meet at the swimming pool.

If you think you don't have anyone like that in your life, perhaps you can find one.

An exercise buddy doesn't need to be a current friend, or even someone you want as a friend. It just needs to be someone who wants to do the same exercise at about the same level as you. You can talk, or not talk. Keep the bar low for qualifying as an exercise buddy. Attendance is the only requirement.

To find an exercise buddy, do the thing you want to do while keeping your eyes peeled for someone else doing the same. Strike up a conversation and at some time mention when you'll be here again. Or your regular time. Maybe they reciprocate with telling you their usual schedule, or maybe you never see them again. If the latter, try again.

There are actually people who say they have enough friends. They tend to be unlikeable people. If you encounter one of these, their rejection is truly all about them, not you.

If you're a beginner, one way to find an exercise buddy is to talk about wanting to start walking, swimming at the Y, swinging through a bucket of balls at the driving range, whatever it is, with co-workers, neighbors, wherever you go. Someone might say 'oh, I always wanted to try that' and then you can see if doing it together works out with both your schedules.

Exercise with a buddy or without one, but doing it with other people can make it easier to stick to a regular schedule and even truly enjoy it.

~ • ~

So these are the three parts to fighting weight gain. There are hundreds of books and articles devoted to these subjects. When all the dust settles, doing what works for you and fits into your lifestyle is what you should do.

Exercise can be integrated into a life that includes watching "The Mentalist" and "So You Think You Can Dance" while babysitting the grandchildren. It doesn't need appointments, changing clothes, or even going outside.

Eating smaller portions with more veggies doesn't need ten whole minutes in the morning to prepare; it can be done by throwing a frozen entre into the briefcase that provides some veggies and daily variety and costs less than the $8 work cafeteria lunch.

It doesn't require following complex and detailed 'half a grapefruit' diets or diving into personal trainer-level exercise. Simply more movement and smaller portions can work. What you do for exercise is totally personal preference. Some is always better than none. Don't let the people who want to sell you things define what exercise is. It's all good.

Hot Flash Medicine

The medical community has a prescription that alleviates hot flashes and reduces osteoporosis, but 70% of doctors flatly refuse to prescribe it. I went to two doctors who refused to prescribe it, and consulted with four others who said they would do the same. Frankly, it damaged my career, something a doctor should never be able to do at whim.

Asking for the medication if you've had the same job for 20 years or don't do public speaking as part of your work simply because you just want to stave off the annoyance, should probably get a 'no' from your doctor. If your husband is running for Senator, or you're the TV nightly news anchor, then yes you must get a prescription. Forcing you to be shamed in public should not be a doctor's choice to make, when he has the medication to prevent it.

~ • ~

The severity of your menopause symptoms is directly related to the suddenness of the hormone change. Find out your family history. A history of mild symptoms means your genetics dictates a gradual tapering off, and if severe symptoms, you are prone to a sudden end.

A wise doctor can help the 'sudden end' folks by providing a gradual tapering off. It doesn't have to be public humiliation; it doesn't have to be torture. That the majority of doctors won't do this is due to a subliminal belief that us women have to pay for the original sin, or something like that. There is no compelling medical reason for not providing a medicinal ramp down. It's just your doctor pushing his weight around.

You might think finding an older woman doctor improves the odds of a ramp down, and perhaps it does, but it's not perfect because that particular woman may have been one of the 30% or so who have a genetic slow ramp down so don't think menopause is a big deal. She never had to lead an all-male meeting looking like she fell in a pool, with sweat drips coming off her hair, drips running down her legs and her wet shirt almost clear and clinging to her bra.

~ ● ~

Combining estrogen and progesterone is effective in reducing long term side effects of taking plain estrogen.

There are progesterone creams that can minimize symptoms, but they often contain far less of the hormone than the labels says. Prescription creams are more trustworthy.

The medical establishment mentions the 'increased' risks of heart attack, stroke, and uterine cancer when taking estrogen. No actual data is presented. It's simply taken for granted that there must be factual evidence because it's said so often. Saying something a lot doesn't make it true. To write this chapter I sleuthed out the actual statistics for the biggest reason behind denying medication that is effective in slowing the progression of osteoporosis, uterine cancer.

The other two, heart attack and stroke, don't need any refuting because their high rate of incidence is due to so many causes and interactions, notably weight and blood pressure, that the effects of medication taken say, ten years prior to the heart attack or stroke can never be shown to be the cause.

Osteoporosis is a bone-weakening condition that results from a long time without estrogen or progesterone. Unlike the slight increases in risk of those other issues, osteoporosis is a 100% occurrence in all women.

No number vagueness there. It happens to every woman, no exceptions. It develops progressively at different rates. But it's inevitable. Slowing down the progression is of significant value to each and every woman.

The main objection to prescribing hormone treatment is the increase in uterine cancer. This cancer results in a mere sliver of the deaths in the US attributable to osteoporosis, and no one says the risk doubles with hormone treatment; it just increases a dinky bit.

To start any discussion on hormone therapy ramifications, know that uterine cancer is uncommon and highly curable. The frequency is small, and grows slightly if you take hormones. The actual numbers are seldom published, because they need to hide the silliness of even mouthing the words.

Anyone who places the risk of uterine cancer right next to osteoporosis and calls them equal has some other agenda, one that has nothing to do with helping menopausal women.

~ • ~

Statistics: To make any sense of medical predictions, understanding the terms related to statistics is needed. Analogies are a useful way to demonstrate what they actually mean.

First off, it's important to have a solid grasp of what 'statistically significant' means. Below that point is called statistically insignificant. Engineering calls it 'in the noise,' meaning in the wavy line that splits A from B.

Because life has so many variables, some of the data points on one side would have gone to the other if the variables combined differently. Science can never be certain of a specific percentage; it assigns a range around that percentage. Changes within that range are not significant.

College kids in math classes learn long and huge calculations for determining statistical significance. The irony is, 98% of the time it boils down to about 3%. Meaning anything that wishes to call itself either an improvement or a detriment must exceed the 3% statistically significant threshold.

When your personal odds change by less than the statistically significant amount, it should not be a factor in any decisions.

Statistical significance doesn't apply to the change, a.k.a. the delta. The delta is a ratio between old instance and new instance.

For instance, if my odds of winning a drawing were 1% and upon buying more tickets are 2%, the delta is that my chances have doubled. The delta is a 100% increase in my chances.

Does that mean I'm a shoo-in to win? I now have 100% better odds. No. My chances are 2%. Doubling my chances, gaining a 100% increase in odds is meaningless unless I know the baseline number, which in this case was 1%. Not 10% or even 40%, which would make doubling my odds something to crow about.

Although the delta is a 100% increase in my odds, that change is still below statistical significance, which is 3%. The baseline change would need to bump to 4% to become statistically significant for me.

When you read about medical studies, often all you get is the delta. Researchers throw the delta around like popcorn at a kid's party but the only statistic that matters is the change from the baseline.

The delta is half a statistic. Whenever an article or report harps on the delta, they are being deceptive.

This is important: whenever a report harps on the delta and does not mention the baseline, they are being deceptive. They are glorifying their research project at the expense of leading people to make huge mistakes. As

Leonard Courtney said, "There are three kinds of lies: lies, damned lies and statistics." The common practice of presenting the delta as if it were the baseline change constitutes statistical lying.

Hypothetically, if my chances of dying are 1.3% with no treatment and 1% with treatment, the delta is a 30% decrease in the risk, so researchers will brag about 30% better odds with treatment. But my personal chances have improved only 0.3%, or one out of 300. Not 90 out of 300, as hearing the delta leads one to believe.

Hearing that my risk decreases 30% with treatment can make me sell my house to afford $200,000 treatment, or even accept horrendous side effects like becoming wheelchair bound. These are not things a sane person would ever do for a 1 in 300 chance.

Back to menopause, if you wonder why a doctor would throw away a chance for a few check-up visits related to medication in return for huge chances of serious injury medical care ten years from now, well, in any other trade it would be called 'job security.'

The risk of uterine cancer is dinky. The best number I could find is that for a woman over 40 the lifetime odds – not ANNUAL odds—of getting uterine cancer are 3% with a survival rate over 92%, and some sites even say 95%. Translated, the annual odds of contracting it are less than 1 in 2,000 but dying of it less than 1 in 28,000. Having this loom large in health decisions makes about as much sense as deciding to stop wearing a seatbelt while living in Kansas because if the car plunges into a body of water the odds of not drowning are 50% better if the driver is seatbelt-free.

Preventing an infrequent bad outcome—drowning in a car— by incurring huge risk during events that are almost certain to happen—fender bender—is not using statistical risk to make a decision; it is disregarding statistical risk entirely. It makes even less sense if your route to work doesn't include a bridge. Or family history of uterine cancer.

Stating that the severity of injury of some fender benders is only a broken nose, so arguing that we should all stop wearing a seatbelt because dying of drowning is worse than a broken nose is a specious argument.

Even if wearing no seatbelt guaranteed 100% odds of escaping from the underwater car, it wouldn't be worth it compared to the downsides.

But even the proponents admit there's a 50% *delta* in the death rate. Meaning if eight out of ten escape now, with two drowning, nine out of ten would escape without a seatbelt on, one drowning. That's a 50% delta. Was two, now is one. Half.

Then, carrying the analogy further, there is no consideration of how many women aren't able to drive anymore due to past auto injuries, or in the case of menopause, are bedridden or in severe pain due to osteoporosis. There's no chance of dying of uterine cancer if the woman dies long before that on the living room rug when she can't get up.

This isn't being flippant; falls are the number one cause of injury-related death in women over 65. Each year, over 200,000 women in the US break a hip due to osteoporosis; fewer than 50,000 are diagnosed with uterine cancer. The 2-year mortality rate due to complications of hip breakage are one in three. This is higher than if every woman who tested positive for uterine cancer died of it. But only 5% do.

Put into real numbers, hip breakage leads to 66,700 deaths per year, while uterine cancer with a 5% mortality rate leads to . . . 2,500 deaths per year.

Of that 2,500, how many can attribute the cancer to taking hormones? Actually, no one can say. It could be ten. Of the hip breakages, how many would be averted if women had the bone mass that hormone treatment would provide? Well, nearly all of them. Making a dent in the progression of osteoporosis is the life-saving part of the equation.

Yet the cancer scare reason is given by doctors today with a straight face. They refuse their patients seatbelts in the spirit of reducing some small amount of one of the many causes of drowning.

Injuries the seatbelt could prevent are dismissed by saying that's only if you get into a fender bender or worse. The almost 100% chance of a fender bender happening in the next thirty years does not seem to matter. He thinks he's preventing drowning, and his attitude towards fender benders is 'don't get in an accident.' Or for older women, the advice is 'don't fall.'

Never, never accept a delta statistic as meaningful. When anyone tells you that the risk goes up 200% if you do X, Y or Z, you need the baseline percentage to make any sense of it.

It's worth considering if the personal chances were 20% and are now 40%, but it's snort-worthy if the chances were .002% and go up to .004%. To be statistically significant the baseline would need to go from 20% to 23%, or 1% to 4%. Going from .01% to 1% does not cross the 3% threshold, even though that's a 10,000% increase.

When a medical statistic is addressing a disease or condition with a frequency in the general population of less than 1 out of 500, it's a safe bet the statistic itself is weak. They didn't collect together enough of a pool of people to crunch the numbers by head count. Rather, it's often the case there was a delta between control group and test group of exactly 1 person.

Medical studies are nearly always done with a rather small group and the results are extrapolated. When the control group is 10,000 and the test group is 10,000, the statistics they spout may be worth considering.

But often the control group is more like 80 and the study group 155! Nearly all medical, psychological, and research studies that take longer than two months have huge participant fallout rate. A study that starts with 155 may have forty people fall out before the end of the study because they move, get some other illness, take other medications that muddy the waters, or just don't want to anymore.

Few products can afford the 1,000 or more participants in twelve states that are really necessary to assign an accurate statistical number. So they run studies with small groups and massage the numbers into statistics that may not, heck, almost NEVER pan out into the real ones in the population at large.

The very reasons that make people fall out of the study, such as taking vitamins or herbal medicines, having other health conditions, poor diet, alcoholism and so on, are in full bloom in the general population.

Many medical studies are performed on groups collected for other reasons: in prisons, college campuses, nursing homes, city neighborhoods.

These results are skewed for reasons like: homogenous age group, homogenous sex, homogenous diet, too many of the same nationality in the group, too many taking the same other medication, and the biggest wildcard, the fallout of those who would actually make the study go the other way.

Pay attention to studies, but if the article talks only about deltas and doesn't contrast the baseline starting point number to the new baseline number, never providing a clue whether your chances of winning the drawing, getting cancer, or drowning in your car surpass the statistical significance number of 3%, then ignore it as researcher bravado.

No one just forgets to mention it if this cure or that prevention surpasses the statistical significance point.

Other drugs:

The jury is in: Black Cohosh doesn't work. Rather, it is effective for the placebo effect only. Which means it works for a few people who really believe it works.

Placebo effect is a very strong force. It's such a strong force that it's the reason for the effectiveness of most folk medicine [yes, effectiveness!], constitutes the value of bad-tasting medicine, and is the reason witch doctors of old could do a dance, light some incense and cure cancer [yes, cure!].

In the US we've done a huge amount of double-blind studies with complex statistical analysis, so can pin a typical number onto the impact of the placebo effect: 30%. When a patient truly believes he or she is receiving effective medicine, it works. Typical anecdotal incidents are like those from WWII when medics, after running out of pain meds, gave beans for pain pills or attached a drip with saline only and said it was morphine, to help wounded soldiers. It diminished the pain for most, but for some it alleviated the pain completely.

Because of the placebo effect's huge efficacy rate, it is worthwhile to dive fully into believing the medicines and vitamins you take will work. But sometimes, as in the case of Over-The-Counter [OTC] menopause medications, they're just taking your money for what is actually 15¢ of inert ingredients.

During double-blind clinical studies on new drugs, the placebo effect is a wild card. For many years the FDA mandated an error in the test setup that resulted in hundreds of high-side-effect, low efficacy drugs being approved. Yes, strange but true.

All drugs need to be tested by double-blind studies for FDA approval. Here's the rub: for many years (no longer I hope!) the patients receiving the inert product during clinical trials truly received inert pills or shots. Now patients who have a problem—they wouldn't be participating if they didn't have the condition being addressed—are obsessed with discerning if they are one of those receiving the real McCoy. When a side effect appears, they believe they are. The side effect could be constipation, stomach upset, dry mouth, skin color changes, dizziness, weird feelings, you name it.

When a person perceives a side effect during a clinical trial, they believe they are on the real drug, so the 30% placebo effect kicks in.

Imagine what the final effect is: a drug that works only 20% of the time but has noticeable side effects will test out as effective 50% of the time, while one with zero side effects but with 40% efficacy will appear to be not as good. Drugs without side effects have a tough time making the grade in clinical trials.

The vast majority of our approved medications have side effects, and there's a reason for that: our very testing method ensures that high-side-effect drugs will receive that 30% bump.

Now some smart doctors realized how placebo effect was affecting the trials so in the 1970s they wanted to provide placebos with a side effect, say a minor stomach upset.

The powers-that-be were up in arms. At the time they FORBID those researchers from ensuring all test subjects experienced side effects if the drug being tested had side effects. I don't know what is standard now; hopefully test integrity has prevailed over hogging all the placebo effect to the real drug, a practice which makes the 'double-blind' into a pane of glass. Providing placebos with side effects is the only way to sort out the truly effective medications from the barely working medications.

Then there's the other thing, the 'people are different' thing. The best example of this is in the antacid medication arena. There are at least four different kinds of non-chewable pill type antacids that are made from entirely different ingredients. They are not variations on a theme. It isn't like a cake, where this recipe calls for one egg and another calls for three, or one uses baking soda and another just salt. These are entirely different ingredients to accomplish the same result. One is cake, one is celery, one is pudding and another is chewing gum, to make an analogy.

For any particular individual, one or two of the antacids work better than the others. Probably because our innards are different or the main cause of our reflux or indigestion varies. Each one works great for 20% of the people taking it and good enough for another 40%.

No one product works for everybody, all the time. There are people, like myself, for whom the top three sellers don't work well but the fourth works wonderfully.

They obviously work for other people or they wouldn't be top sellers. There is such a wide customer base in the antacid market that there's room for four or more products working in entirely different ways to coexist. For any given person maybe two of them work well.

The truth about medicine is almost nothing works 100% of the time. Nothing. When it involves a pill, an injection, or something to drink, if it can work for 30% to 60% of takers, it's good enough to be out there and available. If it works for 90% but kills or injures 2%, it's not for sale. If it works for 60% but causes hospitalization of 0.05% of takers, it's not for sale.

Across all of medicine, if some disinterested party were to make a list of medications that work 95% of the time for everybody, and also have a permanent injury rate of less than 1%, it would be a short list. It would fit on one side of one page. In 14 pt. type. With white space on the bottom half.

Working all the time for everybody isn't the standard we hold for a drug to go on the market. Being a pinch more effective than the placebo effect is our standard.

Drugs that work for more than 30% of people are worth trying when you have that condition. Don't get so married to a single product that you abandon hope if it doesn't work for you. Try one of the others.

Except when it comes to hot flash pills. They don't work. They just want to sell you pills or something for several months, during which time symptoms will diminish anyway, and you'll credit their product for that.

The only standard that makes sense for hot flash fixes is it works significantly within four days or forget it. There is no such thing as a cumulative effect over months for hot flash fixing. They are conning you.

Western medicine professes to be above tapping the well of placebo effect. Don't believe it. The whole aura of authority surrounding doctors is designed to enhance placebo effect.

The pharmacy system, for instance, where only a highly-educated person can hand over your medication after seeing your ID, enhances the placebo effect of every medication. This is not a bad thing. It improves cure rates. That is a good thing.

If I could suggest only one improvement to our medical system, it would be to do more to wring every benefit out of the placebo effect. We could get another 10% bump in effectiveness if our doctors started wearing intimidating face paint, rubbed symbols into the back of our hands, shook rattles near our ears and used incense. OK, I'm joking. A little.

Above the table, western medicine says the only thing that counts are treatments with chemical, scientific, repeatable, double-blind results; below the table, they are working the placebo effect with secret strings.

Don't believe this? Did you know that the best way to improve the efficacy of a medicine is to make a TV commercial plugging it? Right off the bat it's going to have a better efficacy rate for patients who request it because they believe it will work.

Doctors complain that medicines with low efficacy rates are requested by patients, when they would rather prescribe a better-working one.

The problem is, combined with placebo effect that less-good medicine will probably work better for that particular patient. The patient's belief that it will help them carries the water.

Tell or not Tell?

An open letter to every co-worker in the whole world:

You know women of a certain age go through menopause, so if your co-worker with a 23-year-old child suddenly goes very red after you tell a joke, no she hasn't suddenly acquired a prudish streak, and no, she isn't disapproving. She's in menopause.

If you're conducting a meeting and a woman takes off her blazer, don't draw attention by stopping the meeting to pepper her with questions: Is the room too warm? Where's the thermostat? Should I open the door? In fact, regardless of age, ANY time a woman puts on or takes off her sweater or blazer should go without comment. Never comment. It's that easy. Most women will speak their mind if they think the room temperature should be adjusted, and will say it often. Count on it. Simply sliding a sweater on or off, getting red, or shifting in her chair is never a call to action.

Just because you'll never get menopause or it's very far off for you, don't act like I have a psychological condition. It's not in my head. I didn't do it to myself because I got upset or disturbed. Sometimes being in a hot flash is upsetting in itself. It's hard to live with every emotion being punctuated with a physical symptom that I do not control. It doesn't mean I'm overreacting.

If I tell you that I'm in menopause, don't start asking a lot of questions. Go home, or back to your desk and google it. Find your answers there. I'm not your chance to have a thirty minute conversation on menopause. I'm not an expert. I'm just a person who has it.

If you meet a person with a wall-eye, is it appropriate to ask them if everything else is OK, or are there other effects, when did it start, and can't you go to a doctor to get that fixed?

When you meet a bald guy, is it appropriate to launch into the baldness cure you just read about, ask him if he tried any of the potions advertised in internet sidebars, and then ask him how is his wife taking it?

I think not. When I say I'm in menopause, here's the correct response. "Thank you for telling me."

Anything else, look up online later on when I'm not around, and keep it to yourself.

This is hard enough as it is without acquaintances at work making entertainment out of it.

Hide it or Talk About It?

This is a big question. On the one hand, people who care about you should be able to handle being informed and make an accommodation here and there. Things like . . . I need the room to be cooler, I'm going to have compresses in the frig, I'm not going into the sauna or hot tub, don't even ask me to wear the Easter Bunny costume.

If they were on crutches from a sprained ankle, I wouldn't schedule a Parade of Homes tour for us, would I? So they ought to put up with some inconvenience when it's me and it's not a sprained ankle.

On the other hand, menopause is for old people, and I'm not ready. If I don't say a thing maybe no one will ever know. It's a good plan, stoic and brave, except for the getting red and sweaty thing whenever there's a smidge of stress, and forget about a good laugh at a racy joke—I'm going to look upset even if I swear I'm not. I might act odd and not get out of the chair when someone steps into my office, bring two bottles of water to meetings –and chug them both in the course of one meeting.

Letting everyone at work know that I'm going through menopause is a bell that can't be unrung. It may change how younger managers and co-workers view me. I'll be incontrovertibly over-the-hill. For most jobs, though, that scarcely matters.

The downside to not acknowledging it is pretending it's not happening. That might leave me as the only person in the room who thinks nothing is happening. This is also not good for the career.

It would then appear that vanity, not wanting to appear old, makes me pretend it isn't happening, and I want them all to play along. A game of let's pretend. This also doesn't come off well. Rather than make me appear younger and competent, I look like a person who is willing cover up inconvenient facts that don't serve my goals.

My only advice on this is, when you decide, be all in or all out. Doing it halfway doesn't work at all. You can't tell the truth to a few chosen friends but vehemently deny it with other people. It certainly makes sense to wait until a poorly timed hot flash 'outs' you, then concede, yes, it's something I'm going through right now.

Depending upon the severity of symptoms, you may be in the 20% or so who can pull off not mentioning it and no one notices anything. Perhaps you can be one of those who can say, "Oh yes, I went through that eight years ago."

It's a personal decision. Whatever you decide to do, figure out the sentences you wish to say ahead of time. Unprepared, you may blurt out more than you meant to say.

Fade to End

In the first year of menopause, take lots of photos of yourself, or even get professional ones taken. You're going to want these photos when your face starts changing two to five years later.

If you haven't applied face moisturizer daily before menopause, you may wish to start now. It will be a significant factor in reducing the wrinkling and ashiness that will develop over the next few years. When Consumer Reports reviewed several of the special ingredient moisturizers in the $30-$40 price range, their conclusion was that they do make a difference.

They called it tiny, as in hard to discern in a photo, but we live with our faces so it would be huge to us. To put it in perspective, some face lifts end up having a 'tiny' effect, as in some co-workers will think you just had a good night's sleep or freshened up, or perhaps you changed your hairstyle. If a $10,000 facelift has that 'tiny' effect, hand me a pot of that anti-wrinkle moisturizer, please!

~ ● ~

Happiness. Recent studies show there are two paths to happiness. These work for me. I'll share them, and you can make up your own mind.

One: gain experiences, not things. A new couch can seem a fine way to spend money, but three months later will not improve your general level of happiness. Perhaps the only pleasure it really provided was the *experience* of shopping for it and selecting it.

People who love to shop are often not as hot on owning things. New purchases don't find their way out of the bag once it's home, or still has the tags on three weeks later.

Consider adopting a 'catch and release' policy; whatever isn't compelling enough to use within 7 days, return. That way you can have the fun of shopping yet spend the same $100 over and over again.

For the rest of us, if the choice is between a new pair of shoes or a glass of fine wine overlooking a lake at sunset, go for the lake. While my son was growing up, we spent approximately 10% of our income on travel. One could say we lived beneath our means most of the year just to blow the wad in two weeks annually. But now, looking back on our trips to Disneyworld, Yellowstone, Paris, London, New York, Cancun, Niagara Falls, the Grand Canyon and forty other places, what we sacrificed is hard to pinpoint. Nicer dining room set? More shoes? Three winter coats instead of one?

Experiences don't need to be travel. They can be playing miniature golf, going to a movie, taking a cooking class at the local community college, signing up for an activity at the rec center, or getting together with friends. Whatever takes you to a new place, talking to new people, or just enjoying yourself contributes to general happiness for several days.

Even experiences where you don't enjoy yourself, such as being caught in the rain, waiting for a bus running late, or spending the night in an airport are oddly very valuable, because they make you appreciate the little things you take for granted. A raincoat, owning a car, and sleeping in your own bed suddenly become precious and delightful luxuries.

Never underestimate the ability of a totally miserable experience to make you tickled pink happy with ordinary life.

I've seen people forge friendships out of acquaintanceships by sharing their dreadful experience with . . . a vacation, a home repair, a traffic jam, the service at a restaurant. It leads to another story, and another, and pretty soon a bond forms.

Having a great time is nice, but having an awful time is . . . very interesting. If you want to go for the title of most interesting woman in the county, you're going to need some stories. Get out there, take a chance. As I tell my son, things can either go according to plan, or we can have an adventure. Let your adventures begin!

Two: don't compare yourself to how you used to be. Don't hold up that yardstick on how fast and far you used to run, how much you could lift, how you could dig two 3 foot deep holes to plant two trees in the backyard without taking a break. Oh wait, that's me.

Buddhism calls it self-awareness, meditation theory calls it living in the moment, Christianity urges you to awake each morning treating it as a new day. Every religious tradition has similar advice suitable for framing. Really be in today, aware of today, not burdened and saddled and hobbled by past ignominy and yes, even past accomplishments.

I read a story once, written by a woman talking about her father. When he was young, he farmed 80 acres.

When he got older, he cut it back to 20 acres.

In several more years, he cut back to a big garden in the back yard.

Then a small garden.

Now, he was very old. He had a flower box in the window.

He planted and tended that flower box with great enjoyment. When his daughter visited, he told her about the plants and their progress. He planned what he would grow next year.

The flower box gave him joy and feelings of accomplishment. He allowed himself to appreciate what he had today. To passersby, he did a good job; his flowerbox brightened the neighborhood.

Comparing today to the past is just sticking yourself with pins. Life is a process, and this is where you are today.

Would her father be better off if he acutely felt every day that the flowerbox was not worthy, if he couldn't do a big backyard garden then he would do none at all? Is there any value in declaring a certain past accomplishment, body weight, or amount of wrinkles is the only acceptable number and force yourself to feel bad today? Answer: no value at all.

In a cosmic sense, the world does not want you to be unhappy.

People are burdened and put out when they have to deal with other people's grumpiness, issues, feelings of inadequacy, and so on. Going through life, we would rather meet only people who like themselves and don't feel inadequate because they used to do XYZ and now can only do Y.

By being a person who lives as if who they are *today* is who they are, you do me a favor.

A kindness.

By providing that kindness to people you meet today, you atone for the wrongs or mistakes in your past.

It honors the memory of the deceased. If that person ever comforted you when you were sad, or even just told you to knock it off when you were upset, then you know it is their preference that you be happy.

If grief or medical conditions are happening right now, of course you are unhappy right now. This is not about faking being happy or not in pain just to make it easier on others. When your life is difficult, be honest. Grief takes time. We all have spells of worrying about our future.

I'm speaking about people who are troubled by past bad acts, burdened with past mistakes, feeling inadequate because they used to be stronger, richer, prettier, more famous, smarter, more loved. Most people will wear the proverbial hair shirt for the rest of their lives, because to do elsewise would seem to disrespect the importance or devalue the past.

There has to be a way to convince yourself that honoring the past and respecting whatever that was is still fully 100% possible. Inside. Upon request. But today, as a living, breathing human being, it is OK for you to laugh out loud. To live in peace and without preoccupation with the past.

Today I sit in a waiting room with six people; we all converse about weather, the news, the latest gadget on the market, and have a few laughs. I think nothing is amiss with that. I would wish for nothing to be different. It is fine. It is normal. These are normal people, perfectly socially acceptable, and nothing is wrong with this day.

I can't tell that one of them accidentally drove over her toddler 16 years ago and killed him, or one used to own a company employing 90 people and due to a few bad decisions it went bankrupt, or one made a million in a rock and roll band but lost it all to drugs so now manages the store at a golf course, or one told her family her Dad made her executor of his will and left her almost everything, then destroyed the will, or that one was fired for lying on her resume. And one is YOU.

Do these facts need to be present today? Is there any value in my knowing it, if the only consequence of knowing it is to make our little stay in the waiting room uncomfortable?

Is it worthwhile to take past acts and use them as shackles to make today uneasy too?

Is that what God wants? Or for the non-religious, is that a good plan in the greater scheme of things?

If you find yourself thinking, 'those facts must be revealed, it is a lie to interact with anyone while not knowing the worst four things they've ever done in their lives,' you are not accepting that reality is only today. The vast majority of human interaction is based on only who people are today: a store clerk, the next door neighbor, the boss. It is not incumbent upon every person to interact with others based upon their full history, just who they have grown, up to today, into being. And you too, can be who you are today. My favorite saying is, "The mask, given time, becomes the face itself." Pick your mask and wear it well.

Live in the moment. The present is the only tool you have. Find some words or thought that resonates with you so you and I can chat and have a few laughs in the waiting room.

~ • ~

Menopause weight gain is a peculiar thing. I'm a person who maintained the same weight most of my adult life. When I was 53 I could wear clothes I bought at thirty [That reveals I'm not a fashion hound, I suppose]. How attitudes towards eating change after menopause is hard to describe, however, in private polls with several women a few years into menopause. they verify that they attribute much of their weight gain to this attitude change.

In general, it manifests itself as being content with smaller meals but impossible to skip dinner.

I used to be a ballet dancer in my youth, so skipping meals was absolutely normal for me. It's as if 'being hungry' became a state that feels six times worse than it did when I was 25. It isn't, but it is. It's as if the mental justification I used to employ to bear with the hunger no longer works, or no longer resonates with me.

For the first time in my life, the dinner customs of long-lived civilizations make some sense: Japanese, English, Indian, Chinese, French. It is easy to spot that our traditional mealtimes, portions, and the surrounding customs certainly aren't good fits for children, teenagers, mothers of growing children and men, so who was making up these mealtime standards?

Who made these rules, who defined this as 'the proper' way?

Not men; if they had their druthers they would just heap up the main course on their plate and forget the side dishes. Left to their own devices, men would not be stirring a sauce on the stove for fifteen minutes just to make the meat taste a little different.

Men didn't invent casseroles. Neither did women with two kids in diapers.

Now I know; it was menopausal and post-menopausal women. We're the ones who want a little bit of six different things, not just a big heaping plate of macaroni-and-cheese.

We're the ones who think cooked carrots taste better than raw carrots. We're the ones who want the dessert to be after the meal.

We're the ones who invented mashed potatoes and casseroles.

We're the ones who say 'if you want to eat, you're going to sit around the table and talk while you eat my food."

Our adult daughters struggle for 10 or 15 years to master the coordination and find the time to meet our culturally-mandated standards, even as they fall short several times per week. Dinnertime with all those dirty dishes is never how a 25 year old would do it if she had a say in social customs.

If you're observant and have a good memory, it's easy to spot that three sit down meals a day, evenly spaced, are an awful fit for all children [they need to eat five to seven times per day], are almost never what young adults want to do [most would rather have one huge meal and one snack-like meal per day], and a time-suck treadmill for adults between 30 and 45 [they would like one or two no-cook meals per day, a sandwich or fruit].

Every bit of mealtime social customs around the world are tuned to exactly and only how post-menopausal women want it. In this one thing, we rule the world.

You are going to find traditional mealtime customs are more and more attractive to you as you age. This is not because you've become more conservative. It's because those customs have always been finely tuned to what and how and when post-menopausal women want to eat. Breakfast at 7, lunch at noon, dinner at 6. The world runs on your clock now. Finally.

~ ● ~

If you enjoyed this book or found it thought-provoking, please write a review on Amazon!

Getting Through Menopause

http://www.amazon.com/dp/B00N3GZ2CO

www.ingramcontent.com/pod-product-compliance
Lightning Source LLC
Chambersburg PA
CBHW060203290526
45789CB00003B/1136